SOMATIC EXERCISES FOR WEIGHT LOSS

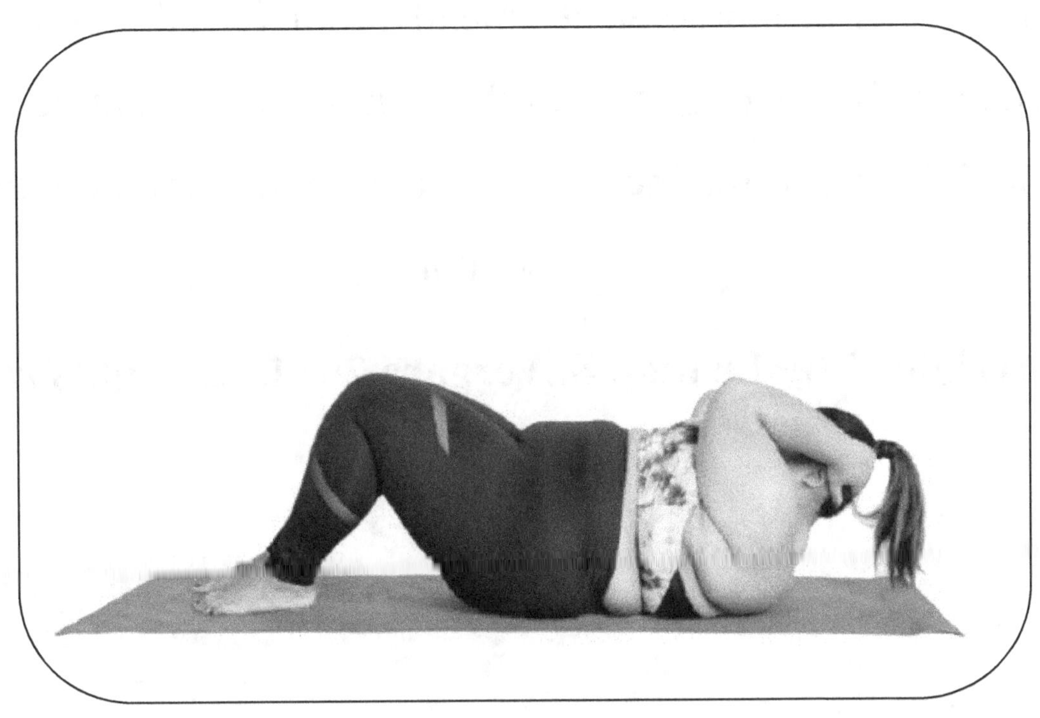

28 Day body Transformation, burn-out excess fat with yoga and increase body flexibility

Lyndon S. Vergara

COPYRIGHT

Before this document is duplicated or reproduced in any manner, the publisher's consent must be gained. Therefore, the contents within can neither be stored electronically, transferred, nor kept in a database. Neither in Part nor full can the document be copied, scanned, faxed, or retained without approval from the publisher or creator.

Copyright © by Lyndon S. Vergara 2024. All rights reserved.

TABLE OF CONTENTS

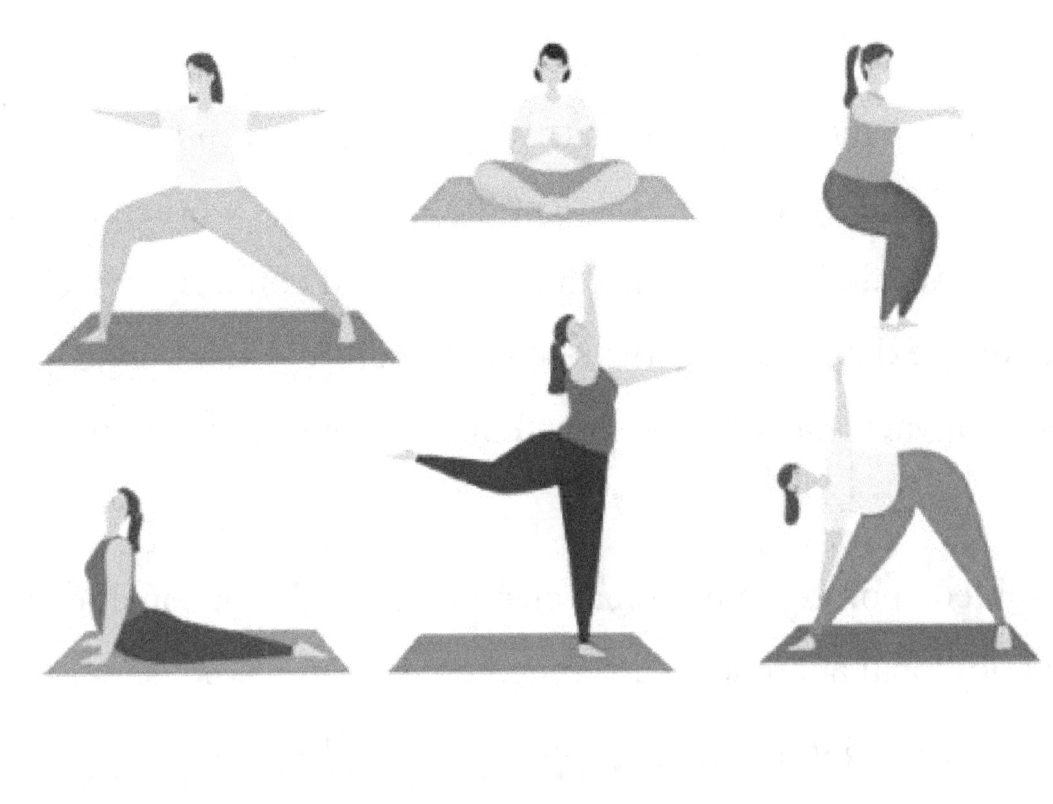

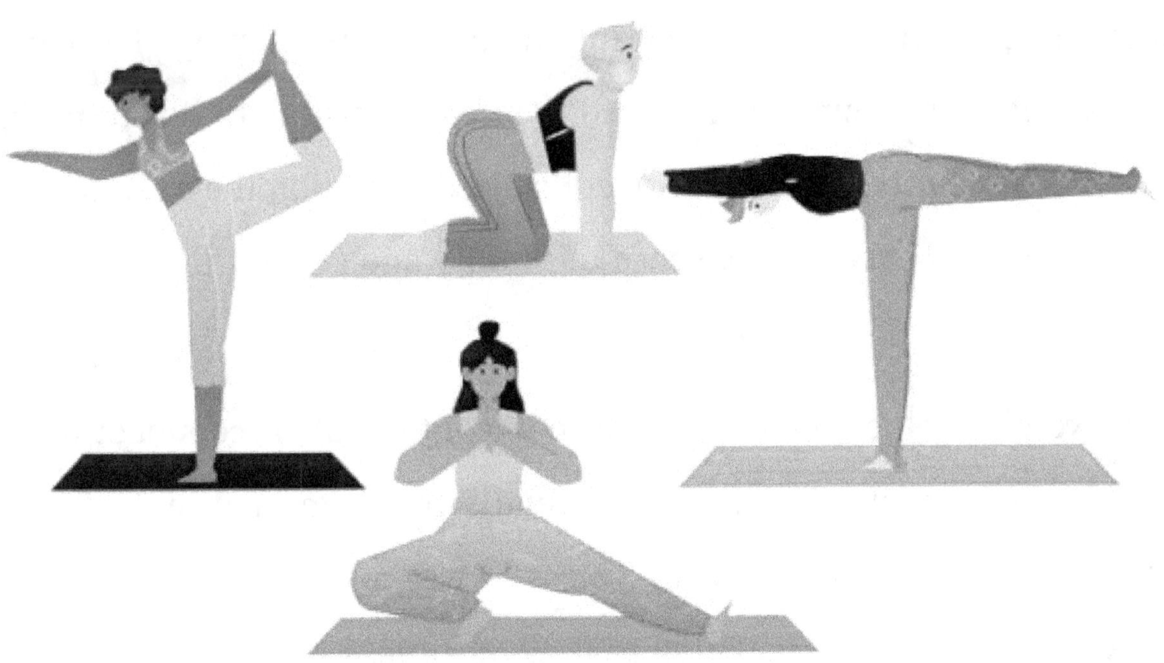

INTRODUCTION

Let me share my story with you. For years, I tried everything to lose weight, fad diets, restrictive meal plans, intense workouts, and even weight loss pills. You name it, I tried it. And while some of these methods worked temporarily, nothing stuck. I would lose a few pounds, but they'd come right back, often leaving me more exhausted and frustrated than before. I felt trapped in an endless cycle, always reaching for something new but never finding what truly worked.

Then, I stumbled upon something that changed everything: somatic exercise. Unlike the traditional approaches I'd relied on, somatic exercise wasn't just about burning calories or pushing my body harder. It was about reconnecting with myself in a whole new way, understanding my body, and allowing movement to be something empowering rather than exhausting. Through gentle, intentional movements, I started to release tension, build strength, and improve my flexibility. To my surprise, I started shedding the excess weight, and more than that, I regained a sense of vitality and control that I hadn't felt in years.

Somatic exercise helped me not only lose weight but also reconnect with my body. I felt stronger, more resilient, and finally free from that feeling of punishment I used to associate with fitness. It was a shift from forcing my body to change to actually listening to it. Over time, I found that I wasn't just "losing weight", I was gaining a better understanding of myself.

In this book, I'll guide you through the practice of somatic exercise and how it can transform your approach to weight loss. You don't need pills, restrictive diets, or high-intensity workouts that leave you drained. Instead, you can learn to move mindfully, rebuild your strength, and feel comfortable in your own skin. Somatic exercise is a journey toward freedom, healing, and lasting change, and I'm here to help you every step of the way.

What is somatic yoga?

Somatic yoga is more than simply a set of poses; it's an internal journey, a practice that invites you to reconnect with yourself in ways that typical workouts and even other types of yoga do not. Imagine moving in such a way that each stretch and movement feels intensely personal, meaningful, and intentional. That is the essence of somatic yoga, finding a rhythm that is uniquely yours, listening to what your body actually requires, and creating an awareness that extends beyond the physical. At its core, somatic yoga integrates traditional yoga concepts with somatic movement, which translates as "of the body." It enables us to become more aware of how our bodies feel on the inside, detecting subtle sensations and learning to release any tension or discomfort we may be holding onto. Rather than following a set of rules or forcing our bodies into tight poses, somatic yoga promotes freedom, flexibility, and, most importantly, self-awareness.

For me, discovering somatic yoga was like finally finding a method to drown out the noise and tension. I learned to move more gently and with intention, and it seemed like my body could finally rest, stretch, and breathe. Unlike previous workouts that left me aching, tight, or weary, somatic yoga was soothing, even contemplative, and unexpectedly effective. With each session, I felt stress melt away, strength increase, and my posture improve without any hard pushing or strain. Somatic yoga invites you to slow down, feel, and connect with your body as it is right now, not forcing it to be what it "should" be, but accepting where you are on this path. Each movement and breath is a time to tune into yourself, to recognize any discomfort or resistance, and to face it compassionately. Over time, this practice helps you gain strength, relieve deeply held tension, and, most importantly, develop trust in your body.

For those of us who have experienced feelings of disconnection from our bodies, cycles of weight loss and gain, injuries, or chronic discomfort, somatic yoga is particularly effective. In addition to helping us lose physical weight, somatic yoga helps us re-establish a connection with our own needs and sensations by emphasizing the interior experience. Somatic yoga is a gradual path to increased strength, flexibility, and inner serenity, helping you to finally feel at ease in your own body. And, in a society where we're often urged to push harder, somatic yoga reminds us that true power comes from listening carefully, moving deliberately, and accepting ourselves exactly as we are.

Why Somatic and Weight loss?

If you're like me, you've probably spent years chasing that elusive "perfect" weight. Maybe you've tried restrictive diets, intense workout programs, or even considered pills or surgeries to speed up the process. And while some of these things may work temporarily, they often leave us feeling drained, disconnected, and sometimes even defeated. I know that struggle because I was there too, constantly fighting with my body, hoping for a magic solution that never came.

But then I learned about somatic exercise, which changed everything. Somatic exercise is more than just moving your body; it is a method to reclaim it, to connect with oneself in a way that feels natural, intuitive, and freeing. Actually, I didn't feel like I was injuring myself by losing weight for the first time. I was beginning to comprehend and even enjoy the way my body moved, identifying and gently releasing tension that had built up over the years. It felt like I was gradually peeling away layers of not only physical weight, but also worry, self-judgment, and dissatisfaction.

So how does somatic exercise help with weight loss? It starts by teaching you to listen. We live in a culture that tells us to push harder, to ignore the body's natural cues of exhaustion or stress. But somatic exercise is different; it encourages us to move mindfully, to feel every part of the body, and to recognize where we're holding onto unnecessary tension. As you practice somatic movements, you gradually rewire how your muscles, joints, and brain communicate. This helps release long-held stress, which, in turn, allows the body to function better, metabolize more efficiently, and let go of stored fat as it naturally recalibrates. Unlike dieting and surgery, somatic weight loss is a gradual process of awareness, healing, and connection. Many people are unaware that being overweight is not just physical, but also emotional and mental. When we carry tension or unresolved emotions, our bodies retain that weight as well. Somatic exercise enables us to move through these experiences, recognizing them and gently letting them go. Each action becomes a step toward eliminating not only pounds, but also the stresses we've been carrying for years.

One of the biggest changes I noticed was in my relationship with food. As I practiced somatic exercise and tuned into my body, I started recognizing when I was truly hungry and when I was eating out of habit, boredom, or stress. The mindful movement practices taught me to respect my body's cues, to savor my meals, and to eat in a way that felt nourishing rather than restrictive. It's amazing how, over time, this practice naturally reshapes your relationship with food without needing a strict diet plan. And the best part? Somatic exercise does not necessitate strong cardiac workouts or strict scheduling. You are not required to push through pain or weariness; instead, you are encouraged to move at your own speed, listening to your body's demands each day. Over time, you develop strength, flexibility, and a greater appreciation for yourself. The weight loss from this path feels sustainable, empowering, and healing because you're no longer fighting your body, but rather working with it.

The benefits of Somatic exercise

If you're reading this, you've probably attempted a number of weight loss procedures that left you feeling exhausted, discouraged, and disconnected from your own body. I've been there, too, the never-ending cycles of diets and workouts that seemed like punishment rather than empowerment. But, for me, somatic exercise has been a game changer. It is not just another fitness fad or quick-fix answer. It's a habit that has completely changed the way I see my body, my health, and even my weight reduction journey.

So, what can somatic exercise do for you? Here are the benefits I experienced, and I hope you find the same sense of relief and transformation:

1. A Deeper Connection with Your Body:

One of the most important benefits of somatic exercise is that it allows you to reconnect with your body. For so long, I felt like I was fighting against myself, trying to lose weight and constantly focusing on what was wrong with me. Somatic exercise helped me change my perspective. Instead of forcing my body to conform to an ideal, I began listening to it, truly listening to what it required. It was the first step toward a healthy connection with myself, after which everything else fell into place. You no longer perceive your body as an enemy, but rather as an ally in your weight loss quest.

2. Reduced Stress and Emotional Healing:

Weight is more than simply a physical concept. I realized that much of the weight I was carrying was not from food, but from worry, anxiety, and unresolved emotions stored in my body. Somatic activities are designed to relieve stress, both physically and emotionally. As I walked attentively through each session, I began to release the stress that had built up over the years. That release not only feels nice, but it also makes space for healing. When you are not carrying mental weight, it is simpler to lose physical weight as well.

3. Improved Strength and Flexibility:

Unlike brutal gym workouts that require you to push through pain or weariness, somatic exercise allows you to build strength gradually, gently, and with full-body awareness. I was surprised to discover that with time, not only did I get more flexible, but also stronger. The moderate movements helped release muscle tension, and as I stretched and strengthened my body, I felt a renewed sense of life. Weight loss occurs as a result of increased strength and mobility. When you feel powerful, you are more inclined to take proper care of your body, which shows in how you look and feel.

4. Better Posture and Body Awareness:

For years, I had no idea how much tension I was harboring in my body. Poor posture, sagging shoulders, tense hips, all of this compounded up over time. Somatic exercise is about learning to move with ease and releasing tension. As I became more aware of how I was carrying myself, my posture improved. When your body moves with ease and balance, it burns energy more efficiently, and you naturally begin to lose weight. What is the best part? It also makes you feel more comfortable in your own flesh.

5. Sustainable and Gentle Weight Loss:

This is the moment that genuinely altered the game for me. Somatic exercise isn't about harsh diets or workouts; it's about making long-term changes. You do not need to starve yourself or put in endless hours of exercise. Weight loss with somatic exercise occurs spontaneously since it is associated with self-care and self-awareness. Weight reduction comes naturally when you treat your body with care, accept its needs, and let go of past patterns of restriction or punishment. Furthermore, because it takes a soft, holistic approach, the outcomes are more long-lasting and gentler on your body.

6. Increased Energy and Vitality:

I used to feel sluggish, fatigued, and dejected at the end of the day, even after attempting to "stay active" with strenuous exercise. Even after a gentle session, somatic exercise left me feeling more energized. This is because somatic activity helps your body work optimally, it supports metabolism, enhances circulation, and increases overall energy. When you're energized, you naturally move more, make better decisions, and live your life in a way that promotes health and well-being.

7.   A Compassionate, Non-Judgmental Approach:

Finally, and maybe most crucially, somatic exercise fosters compassion. It does not encourage you to move faster, do more, or be someone you are not. It encourages you to go at your own pace, respecting where you are and what your body requires at the time. This nonjudgmental attitude to movement and weight loss was the catalyst I needed to quit being so hard on myself. It helped me stop comparing myself to others and instead focus on my own healing. It serves as a reminder that this is your path, at your own pace, and that's what matters most.

These are the benefits of somatic exercise that I have received, and I am confident that you will experience the same. If you're weary of feeling detached from your body, exhausted by rigorous diets and workouts, or simply overwhelmed by the weight loss path, somatic exercise offers a quiet, comprehensive solution.

CHAPTER 1: SOMATIC EXERCISE FOR STRESS RELIEF

How Somatic Movements Calm the Mind and Body

Somatic movements are more than just physical exercises; they explore the profound relationship between the body and the mind. In a world where stress appears to be an unavoidable part of our everyday lives, it's easy to underestimate how profoundly tension may develop in the body. This strain manifests itself not only physically, but also emotionally and mentally.

Somatic exercises are fundamentally meant to help you release tension and reconnect with your body in a way that helps both your mind and body to achieve balance, peace, and relaxation. You might be wondering how somatic movements relax the mind and body. The approach is founded on a fundamental principle: awareness. Somatic exercises focus on the body's sensations, allowing you to become more aware of how you move, breathe, and hold yourself.

This awareness draws attention away from the chaotic, stress-inducing thoughts that frequently race through our minds. In some ways, these activities help you focus on the present moment, allowing tension and worry to slip away from you.

Understanding the Mind-Body Connection

Stress doesn't just sit in our heads; it often manifests in our bodies. Whether it's tight shoulders, clenched jaws, shallow breathing, or a racing heartbeat, these are all signs that your body is holding onto stress. If left unchecked, this physical manifestation of stress can lead to chronic pain, fatigue, and other health issues. Somatic movements are incredibly effective in reversing this cycle. Think of somatic exercises like a reset button. The slow, mindful movements engage the body's parasympathetic nervous system, often referred to as the "rest and digest" system. When this system is activated, it counters the "fight or flight" response, lowering your heart rate, reducing muscle tension, and calming your breath. As you move through these exercises, your body learns how to soften, how to release the tightness that stress has built up over time.

Mindful Movement: Letting Go of Emotional Stress

When we move deliberately, we direct our attention to the sensations we are feeling, such as the feel of the floor beneath our feet or the stretch in our muscles. This form of awareness can also help us release deep-seated emotional strain. Many of us store emotional stress in specific places of our bodies, such as chest tightness from anxiety or neck stiffness from overthinking. Somatic exercises target these areas with gentle stretches, motions, and even breathwork, urging the body to release whatever it is holding onto.

For example, consider movements like body scanning, where you slowly move your attention through each part of your body, noticing tension and consciously deciding to release it. Over time, as you practice these exercises, you create new neural pathways that associate movement with relaxation rather than stress. This transforms your body's natural response to stress, making it easier to calm down and reduce tension when life gets overwhelming.

A Holistic Approach to Stress Relief

It's also worth noting that somatic exercises can help you prevent stress rather than just manage it. By incorporating these exercises into your regular routine, you will develop the habit of listening to your body before stress arises. Somatic exercises, like checking in with your thoughts or emotions on a regular basis, offer a physical practice for checking in with your body. This continual focus on body-mind balance keeps you grounded, making it less likely that you'll be overwhelmed by the challenges of ordinary life. When we're calmer and more at peace, we can make better decisions, including those affecting our health. Somatic exercises promote a good mind-body connection, which can lead to better habits such as more conscious eating and a greater inclination to participate in physical activity. This can help with weight loss not by driving the body into drastic measures, but by aligning it with a state of wellness in which movement is enjoyable rather than stressful.

Somatic Movement for Weight Loss and Beyond

For people aiming to reduce weight, somatic motions might be an important element of the process. While these exercises do not need significant cardio or strength training, they do help you reconnect with your body in fundamental ways. Reducing stress and tension allows your body to perform more efficiently, which improves digestion, boosts energy levels, and stabilizes mental well-being. This holistic approach to health, which emphasizes relaxation and self-care, makes weight loss a natural outcome of general well-being.

Remember that the goal is more than just "burning calories" or "shedding pounds." It is about developing a relationship with your body based on respect, compassion, and mindfulness. Somatic exercises teach you to move in a way that feels good, not forced. As you progress, you may find yourself moving with more ease and confidence, naturally leading to a healthier body.

Using Somatic Practices to Reduce Daily Stress

If you've ever felt overwhelmed by the stresses of daily life, whether it's balancing job, family, or personal difficulties, you're not alone. Stress can feel like a constant companion, and it typically makes everything more difficult, including maintaining your health and weight. You may notice that stress influences your food patterns, energy levels, and overall sense of well-being. It can also cause weight gain or make it more difficult to shed weight since your body stores stress in physical ways.

However, the good news is that somatic practices, or body-focused, mindful movements, can be a very powerful tool for lowering stress. These techniques can help you relax and re-establish a connection with your body, providing a road to both mental and physical well-being.

- **Start Where You Are: Reconnecting with Your Body:**

It can be easy to forget how tightly your body holds onto stress, especially when you're constantly on the go. But somatic practices remind us that the body speaks to us, and it's often trying to tell us that we're carrying more than we realize. Think about the tightness you feel in your shoulders after a long, stressful day, or the way your neck feels stiff when you're anxious. These are signals from your body, asking you to slow down and pay attention. One of the simplest ways to use somatic practices to reduce stress is to start by checking in with yourself. Take a few minutes each day to pause and scan your body, noticing areas of tension or discomfort. This is the first step in understanding how stress shows up in your body. Somatic exercises like gentle stretching, breathing techniques, or simple body movements can help you release this tension, creating space for relaxation.

For example, you can try a basic movement like shoulder rolls, which include slowly and gently lifting your shoulders towards your ears and then rolling them back and down, letting go of whatever tension you may be harboring. As you do this, take deep breaths and let your breath drive your movement. The act of focusing on your body, along with exercise, can help reset your nervous system, minimizing the physical impacts of stress and restoring you to a more grounded condition.

- **Slow, Mindful Movements for Stress Reduction:**

Another key benefit of somatic practices is that they encourage a slower, more mindful approach to movement. Often, when we're stressed, we move quickly, reacting to the pressures around us without thinking. This fast-paced movement can heighten our feelings of anxiety and stress. Somatic exercises invite us to slow down, to move with purpose, and to listen to our bodies. Gentle, flowing movements, such as a slow, intentional stretching practice or yoga-inspired motions, can engage the parasympathetic nerve system (the "rest and digest" system), which helps to regulate the body's stress response. In these moments, you are allowing your body to relax rather than be always awake.

This is not about straining your physical boundaries or striking beautiful positions. It's about becoming aware of how your body feels during each movement and allowing yourself to be there without judgment. As you begin to include these mindful movements into your everyday routine, you will notice that your body opens up, becomes more relaxed, and balanced. Your stress reaction gradually becomes less reactive, and your body learns to deal with life's obstacles more calmly.

- **Using Breath to Calm the Mind and Body:**

One of the simplest yet most powerful somatic practices is breathing. Our breath has an incredible ability to influence our nervous system, and deep, mindful breathing is a tool you can use to reduce stress any time of day.

When you're feeling overwhelmed, your breath often becomes shallow and quick. This can keep you stuck in a stressed state. But by consciously slowing your breath, you signal to your body that it's time to relax. Practice deep breathing techniques by inhaling slowly for a count of four, holding for a moment, and then exhaling for a count of six or eight. Focus on how your chest and belly rise and fall with each breath.

Even just five minutes of focused breathing can help reduce the physical tension you're holding in your body, lower your heart rate, and calm your mind. This is a practice you can do anywhere, at your desk, in your car, or at home. Over time, as you become more comfortable with your breath, it can become a powerful anchor for reducing stress throughout the day.

- **Making Somatic Practices Part of Your Daily Routine**

The beauty of somatic practices is that they don't require a special class or expensive equipment. You don't need to set aside hours for long workouts. Five to ten minutes a day can be enough to start reaping the benefits. Incorporating somatic practices into your daily routine might look like:

- spending some time stretching gently and checking in with your body in the morning or before bed.

- Taking deep breaths while waiting for the bus or when seated at your desk.

- allowing your body to release any stress by taking thoughtful breaks during the day to stand up, stretch, or go for a walk.

You'll notice a change when you start incorporating these techniques. You'll feel more in control of how your body reacts to stress and it won't feel so overpowering. Your weight reduction strategy will benefit from this serenity and stress relief as well. You make better decisions when your body is less stressed; eating becomes more attentive, and moving becomes more pleasurable rather than just another chore on your to-do list.

CHAPTER 2: SOMATIC EXERCISE FOR PAIN AND WEIGHT LOSS MANAGEMENT

Using Somatic Practices to Manage Pain and Improve Mobility

If you have been dealing with chronic pain, such as joint pain, muscular tightness, or back pain, you are aware of how restricting it may be. Not only can pain impact your physical health, but it also has an impact on your motivation, mood, and capacity to completely enjoy life. It can even make it more difficult to exercise or move, which can lead to a vicious cycle where the less you move, the greater the pain is. Furthermore, this pain might become considerably more excruciating if you are carrying excess weight. The good news is that somatic practices can be an effective way to support your general health and weight loss journey while also helping you manage pain and increase your mobility.

I want to talk to you because I understand how frustrating it is to feel like your discomfort prevents you from moving freely. I know how easily it may make you feel defeated. An alternative perspective on pain is provided by somatic practices, which emphasize thoughtful, gentle movements that help you listen to your body, let go of stress, and progressively regain your strength and mobility. The goal of these motions is to learn how to move in a way that feels secure, supported, and healing rather than to force through pain.

- **Understanding How Somatic Practices Can Help with Pain:**

The concept of bodily awareness lies at the heart of somatic activities. It's simple to lose touch with our body while we're in pain, either because we're preoccupied with the agony or because we choose not to move at all. Slowing down, focusing, and increasing your awareness of your body's sensations in space are all encouraged by somatic exercises. You can start to pinpoint the movement patterns that are causing your discomfort by focusing this awareness on the places where you experience pain.

Somatic activities, for instance, may assist you in recognizing that you frequently overcompensate with your hips or shoulders when moving if you suffer from lower back pain. You can begin to alter your posture and relieve needless stress by performing particular motions that are intended to raise awareness of these regions. This may eventually result in better body alignment and pain reduction.

Somatic activities are soft and thoughtful, promoting slow and controlled motions that assist the body relearn how to move without aggravating discomfort, in contrast to high-intensity exercises that can strain your muscles. These exercises aid in the release of deep-seated muscle tension, enhance flexibility, and help you regain your body's equilibrium, all of which are critical for pain management.

- **Gradually Restoring Mobility Through Somatic Movement:**

The ability of somatic activities to gradually help you regain mobility, even if you've been struggling with stiffness or limited movement for a while, is one of their most lovely features. It's simple to become rigid and less flexible when discomfort restricts your range of motion. But with somatic exercises, you can gently stretch and strengthen your body, overcoming the resistance and rigidity brought on by pain.

You might begin with easy exercises like rolls or mild stretches, paying attention to your breathing as you go. These motions promote blood flow, relieve tense muscles, and progressively regain range of motion. You don't have to push yourself too hard or too quickly with somatic activities because they may be tailored to your existing level of mobility. Start with modest, easy motions and increase as your body permits.

You'll discover that you may start moving more easily as your mobility increases. This will facilitate your participation in other weight-loss-promoting activities, such swimming, walking, or mild aerobic workouts. Knowing that your body is progressively developing the flexibility it needs to move more comfortably will give you a sense of empowerment with every tiny accomplishment, whether it be standing a bit taller, bending a little deeper, or stretching a little farther.

- **Building Strength and Confidence:**

Somatic practices also focus on rebuilding strength in a way that is compassionate and gradual. If you've been avoiding certain movements because they cause pain, you might feel hesitant to try again. But somatic exercises help you build strength through controlled, low-impact movements, strengthening muscles in a balanced way that doesn't overwhelm the body. This gradual strength-building process not only helps alleviate pain but also gives you the confidence to take on more physical activities over time.

For example, practices like somatic bodyweight exercises, where you focus on slow, mindful movements to engage different muscle groups, can help strengthen muscles around the joints, which in turn supports better mobility and less pain. Over time, these exercises help create a solid foundation of strength and stability, which is essential for overall health and weight management.

Pain Management and Weight Loss: A Symbiotic Relationship

It's vital to understand that pain relief and weight loss frequently go hand in hand. When you're in discomfort, it's natural to feel less inclined to move, which can lead to weight gain or make weight loss seem difficult. Somatic techniques stop the pattern by pushing you to move in ways that feel pleasurable, rather than painful. As your pain and mobility improve, you'll feel more capable of engaging in physical exercise, which can contribute to healthier weight management. Somatic activities also help to minimize the emotional impact of chronic pain on your mental health. Pain can create tension, irritation, and even sadness, which can result in poor eating habits or a lack of motivation. By minimizing pain through mindful exercise, you can also enhance your mental health, resulting in a positive feedback loop that promotes weight reduction and overall health.

- **Moving with Compassion and Patience:**

Above all, embrace somatic techniques with patience and compassion for oneself. Healing is a journey, not a race. As you do somatic exercises, take the time to appreciate your body's current state and acknowledge any little improvements. If you can move more freely, feel less pain, or regain strength, those are triumphs worth celebrating.

Somatic activities do not include pushing through discomfort or accomplishing a specific fitness goal. They emphasize movement in unison with your body, knowing its demands, and respecting its limitations. With constant practice, you will not only observe changes in your pain and mobility, but also feel more free and confident in your body.

How Somatic Movements Aid in Weight Loss by Alleviating Chronic Pain

Dealing with chronic pain is more than simply a physical hardship; it may be emotionally tiring, psychologically draining, and frequently depressing. If you've been carrying additional weight while simultaneously dealing with pain in your joints, back, or muscles, you know how tough it can be to find the energy and drive to exercise. Pain can limit not only your physical movement but also your capacity to perceive a path forward. I absolutely understand the experience; it's easy to feel trapped by both pain and weight, as if they're two huge things you can't shake. But here's the good news: somatic motions can help interrupt the pattern.

Somatic movements not only improve your physical well-being by relieving chronic pain and increasing mobility, but they can also pave the road for empowered and lasting weight loss. The goal is to learn how these techniques gently relieve stress, increase circulation, and build a healthier relationship with your body.

- **Reducing Pain, Increasing Mobility, and Reigniting Motivation:**

Chronic pain causes more than just discomfort. Pain typically results in a lack of motivation to move. When you avoid physical activity due to pain, it can lead to weight gain, making the pattern even more difficult to break. Somatic exercises, with their gentle, thoughtful approach, can help you progressively reduce pain and enhance mobility, allowing you to move more.

Think of somatic movements like a bridge, helping you transition from a place of pain and immobility to one of increased freedom and comfort. These movements are designed to release the tension that's often held in muscles, joints, and connective tissues due to chronic pain. As this tension eases, you'll find that your range of motion improves, making it easier to move, exercise, and eventually engage in activities that can support weight loss, like walking or low-impact aerobic exercises.

- **Alleviating Pain to Unlock Energy for Movement:**

Pain is taxing, both physically and emotionally. When you're continually in pain, it's quite difficult to muster the energy and determination to exercise. This is where somatic motions excel. Because they emphasize slow, controlled, and attentive motions, they do not increase the body's stress level. Instead, they induce modest tension releases, which provide relief.

By actively participating in somatic exercises, even at a slow speed, you can help your muscles, joints, and fascia (the connective tissue that surrounds your muscles) relax. When the pain begins to subside, you may be startled by the amount of energy that returns. This energy is essential for moving more, which increases the probability of weight loss.

For example, simple movements like hip circles or shoulder rolls help to mobilize tight areas and increase blood flow to your muscles and joints. As these areas loosen up, you'll likely feel less pain, and more importantly, you'll feel more energized and willing to move further. This can be the starting point for gradually increasing your activity level, creating a positive feedback loop where less pain equals more movement, which eventually leads to better health and weight management.

- **Boosting Circulation and Metabolism:**

Chronic pain can sometimes lead to poor circulation and a sluggish metabolism, making it even harder for your body to burn calories or recover from exercise. Somatic movements help by improving blood flow and oxygenation to your muscles and tissues, which boosts circulation. Improved circulation also helps your body's natural healing process by reducing inflammation and tension, which are often contributors to chronic pain.

As blood flow increases, your metabolism may improve, allowing your body to function more efficiently. This can have a direct impact on weight loss, as an efficient metabolism helps burn calories more effectively. The more often you practice somatic movements, the more you're likely to see a shift in how your body handles energy and weight. Instead of feeling like your body is "fighting" against you, somatic practices help you restore balance and support the natural processes that allow for weight loss.

- **Releasing Emotional Tension: The Hidden Link Between Pain and Weight:**

It's also vital to understand that chronic pain and emotional stress are frequently linked. When you're in physical pain, the emotional toll can be severe - irritation, anxiety, and even melancholy might arise. These emotions, in turn, might influence your eating patterns, making it difficult to make good decisions or stay inspired to exercise.

Somatic techniques promote a mind-body connection, helping you to become aware of emotional stress held in your body. This emotional stress frequently manifests itself in the shoulders, neck, or back, contributing to both pain and poor coping techniques such as overeating or emotional eating.

By using somatic movements, you can start to release not just physical tension but also emotional stress. For example, gentle stretching combined with focused breathing can help ease both mental and physical tension. As you release these emotional blocks, your body becomes more open, not just physically but emotionally, making it easier to make healthier choices and stay consistent with your weight loss goals. This emotional release is crucial in managing chronic pain and supporting long-term well-being.

- **Moving with Compassion and Patience:**

As you incorporate somatic movements into your routine, it's important to remember that the process of healing, improving mobility, and losing weight is gradual. The key is not pushing your body too hard, but rather listening to it and moving with patience and compassion. Healing takes time, and somatic exercises are about honoring your body's pace.

The focus is on progress, not perfection. Every small, mindful movement you make is a step toward less pain, greater mobility, and eventual weight loss. Be kind to yourself as you take these steps, knowing that each one is helping you move toward a healthier, more comfortable body.

- **Somatic Movements: Part of a Balanced Weight Loss Journey**

It's also worth emphasizing that, while somatic movements are an effective technique for pain management and mobility improvement, they can complement other types of movement and healthy behaviors. As your pain subsides and your mobility improves, you'll feel more capable of participating in other activities such as walking, swimming, or strength training. These, together with a well-balanced diet and mindful eating, form a sustainable and humane weight loss strategy.

CHAPTER 3: SOMATIC BREATH AND VISUALIZATION EXERCISES

How the Somatic Breathing Techniques Support Weight Loss

You're not alone if your weight loss journey has ever left you feeling overburdened, nervous, or just stuck. Feelings of anger, remorse, and even self-doubt can arise when you struggle to lose weight. However, the truth is that your body's response to stress and weight is greatly influenced by your breathing. The best part is that you may use somatic breathing techniques to help you harness your body's innate healing, relaxation, and weight loss capabilities.

It's simple to concentrate on the physical components of weight loss, such as exercise, diets, and calorie tracking. But we frequently ignore the mind-body link, which is another important factor. One of the most effective tools you have for maintaining mental and physical balance is your breath, which may help you manage stress, control your emotions, and speed up your metabolism. A subtle yet effective method of gaining these advantages is through somatic breathing exercises.

It's simple to concentrate on the physical components of weight loss, such as exercise, diets, and calorie tracking. But we frequently ignore the mind-body link, which is another important factor. One of the most effective tools you have for maintaining mental and physical balance is your breath, which may help you manage stress, control your emotions, and speed up your metabolism. A subtle yet effective method of gaining these advantages is through somatic breathing exercises.

The Link Between Stress, Breathing, and Weight

Understanding the connection between stress, breath, and weight is crucial before delving into the mechanics of somatic breathing. Stress causes us to breathe shallowly, frequently into our chests, which triggers the body's "fight or flight" reaction. Stress chemicals like cortisol, which have been connected to weight gain, especially around the abdomen, may be released as a result. Shallow breathing and ongoing stress can eventually interfere with your metabolism and make weight loss more difficult.

On the other hand, deep, attentive breathing might have the opposite impact, lowering cortisol levels, calming your nervous system, and promoting fat loss. By practicing somatic breathing, you're inhaling intentionally rather than just to survive, which helps your body feel more relaxed, balanced, and in harmony with your weight loss objectives.

Somatic Breathing and Its Role in Weight Loss

Somatic breathing is all about awareness and conscious connection to your breath and body. It's not just about inhaling and exhaling, it's about bringing your awareness to the rhythm and depth of your breath, feeling how it moves through your body, and using it to release tension. Through somatic techniques, you can begin to breathe more fully, more deeply, and with more intention, which directly supports your weight loss journey.

Here are a few ways somatic breathing can support weight loss:

- Stress Reduction: As mentioned, when you're under stress, it can lead to overeating or cravings, especially for comfort foods. Somatic breathing helps you activate your body's relaxation response, which counters stress and helps reduce emotional eating. By incorporating breathing exercises into your day, you can lower your stress levels, decrease cortisol, and create a sense of calm that encourages more mindful eating habits.

- Improved Digestion: Stress doesn't just affect your mood — it can impact your digestion too. Shallow breathing or holding your breath under stress can slow down your digestive system, making it harder for your body to process food and absorb nutrients effectively. On the other hand, deep belly breathing (diaphragmatic breathing) encourages better blood flow to your digestive organs, helping to promote healthy digestion and absorption. This can support your body in utilizing nutrients more efficiently, which may help with weight management.

- Increased Oxygen and Energy: When you practice somatic breathing, you increase the oxygen supply to your cells, helping your body's metabolic processes run more efficiently. With improved oxygenation, you'll feel more energized, and that boost in energy can help motivate you to move more, engage in physical activity, and continue with your weight loss efforts.

- Releasing Tension: Chronic tension in the body, often from stress or emotional baggage, can physically block energy flow and hinder your body's ability to function optimally. Through somatic breathing, you can actively release tension in areas that may hold onto emotional or physical stress, areas like the belly, hips, shoulders, and chest. As you release this tension, your body will feel more open, and it will be easier for you to engage in exercise, eat mindfully, and make better choices that support your weight loss goals.

- Mindful Awareness and Emotional Balance: Somatic breathing connects the mind and body. By focusing on your breath, you create a space for awareness. awareness of your body, your emotions, and your cravings. For those who turn to food for comfort or as a way to cope with stress, breathing techniques can provide a way to pause, reflect, and choose a more balanced response. Instead of reacting to emotions by reaching for food, somatic breathing can give you a moment to process your emotions in a healthy way.

Practical Somatic Breathing Techniques for Weight Loss

If you're ready to incorporate somatic breathing into your daily routine, here are a few simple techniques to get started:

1. **Diaphragmatic Breathing (Belly Breathing):**

   - Sit or lie down in a comfortable position.

   - Place one hand on your belly and the other on your chest.

   - Take a slow, deep breath in through your nose, expanding your belly outward as you inhale. Make sure your chest stays still.

   - Exhale slowly through your mouth, feeling your belly fall back toward your spine.

   - Repeat for 5–10 minutes, focusing on the rise and fall of your belly with each breath.

2. **This technique activates the parasympathetic nervous system,** promoting relaxation and stress relief. It also helps increase oxygen flow to the body, aiding digestion and metabolism.

3. **4-7-8 Breathing:**

   - Inhale deeply through your nose for a count of 4.

- Hold the breath for a count of 7.

  - Exhale slowly through your mouth for a count of 8.

  - Repeat for 4–6 cycles.

4. This breathing technique helps calm your mind and regulate your emotional state, reducing stress and promoting balance.

5. **Box Breathing**:

  - Inhale for 4 counts.

  - Hold your breath for 4 counts.

  - Exhale for 4 counts.

  - Hold your breath again for 4 counts.

  - Repeat for several cycles.

6. Box breathing helps regulate the nervous system, reduce anxiety, and create a sense of calm. It's great for moments when you feel stressed or overwhelmed, which can help you avoid emotional eating and cravings.

Integrating Somatic Breathing into Your Weight Loss Journey:

How to Include Somatic Breathing in Your Weight Loss Process

It doesn't need to be difficult or time-consuming to incorporate somatic breathing into your weight loss regimen. Start with only a few minutes every day, whether it's to wind down in the evening or to establish a peaceful tone for the day in the morning. You'll eventually see how mindful breathing promotes improved digestion, healthier nutrition, and a more stable emotional state in addition to helping you manage stress.

Using somatic breathing techniques gives your body the resources it needs to heal itself. It's about developing a more positive, healthy relationship with your body, where losing weight is about promoting and nourishing your body's natural functions rather than about fighting for it. Breathing exercises can be a very effective ally in your weight reduction journey if you have the patience, perseverance, and self-compassion to use them.

Using the Mind-Body Connection to Achieve Your Weight Loss Goals

You may feel like your body and mind are against you if you're having trouble losing weight. Despite your best efforts, it might be discouraging to not see progress. The reality is that the mind and body are intricately linked, and when you align them, losing weight becomes easier, more satisfying, and more sustainable.

When we consider weight loss, we frequently just consider outward behaviors like exercise, calorie counting, and dietary choices. Naturally, these are significant, but they only deal with a portion of the problem. How you relate to your body and how you behave are greatly influenced by your thoughts, feelings, beliefs, and mentality. You can open up new options for healing and weight loss that may seem unattainable at the moment by fortifying the mind-body connection.

The Power of Your Mind in Shaping Your Body:

It's easy to think of the body as a separate entity from the mind, but they are in constant communication. Your thoughts influence your physical state, and your body's condition can affect your emotional and mental state. When you are stressed, your body tenses up. When you feel happy or relaxed, your body responds with ease. This constant feedback loop is a powerful tool you can use to support your weight loss goals.

When we feel overwhelmed or discouraged, it's easy for the mind to slip into negative patterns of thinking: "I'll never lose this weight," "I'm just not disciplined enough," or "This is too hard." These thoughts create emotional stress, which can manifest in physical tension or cravings, making it harder to stick to healthy habits. The mind can become a barrier to your progress.

But here's the good news: You can rewire your thoughts to help your body repair in a healthy way. By strengthening your mind-body connection, you may change your emotional state, overcome negative thought patterns, and cultivate a sense of empowerment and self-compassion, which will help you lose weight.

How the Mind-Body Connection Supports Weight Loss:

- Changing Your Relationship with Food

Many people struggle with emotional eating, using food to cope with stress, anxiety, or even boredom. When your mind is disconnected from your body, it's easy to fall into these patterns without realizing it. Mind-body awareness helps you become more mindful of your body's signals, so you can differentiate between true physical hunger and emotional cravings.

When you start paying attention to how your body feels before, during, and after eating, you begin to make more conscious decisions. Mindful eating, which comes from a strong mind-body connection, allows you to savor your food, listen to your hunger cues, and stop when you're full. This prevents overeating and helps you develop a healthier relationship with food — not as a source of comfort, but as fuel for your body.

- Breaking the Cycle of Stress and Emotional Eating

Stress is a powerful force in our lives, and it often leads to emotional eating. You may have experienced a situation where, after a stressful day, you found yourself reaching for a sugary snack or a bowl of comfort food. The mind can easily use food as a way to cope with stress, but this habit can derail weight loss goals and create feelings of guilt.

By using the mind-body connection, you can interrupt this cycle. When stress arises, instead of turning to food, you can use mindfulness techniques to focus on your breath, notice where tension is stored in your body, and consciously relax. Practicing somatic breathing exercises and body awareness can ground you in the present moment, helping you manage stress without needing to rely on food for comfort.

- Cultivating a Growth Mindset

Weight loss, like any personal goal, involves ups and downs. Some days, progress will be visible, and other days, it might feel slow or even nonexistent. The key to staying on track is developing a growth mindset, the belief that challenges and setbacks are a natural part of the process, not a reflection of your worth or capabilities.

By connecting with your body, you can start to recognize that your body is on your side. Every step, no matter how small, is progress. Being kind to yourself and practicing patience, especially when things feel tough, helps maintain your motivation and belief in your ability to succeed.

The mind-body connection also helps you see weight loss as a journey, not a destination. It shifts the focus from short-term results to the long-term goal of health and well-being. This shift in perspective is crucial for creating lasting change and avoiding the frustration that comes from striving for quick fixes.

- Understanding Your Body's Signals

Your body has incredible wisdom, but sometimes we are too disconnected from it to truly understand what it needs. The mind-body connection helps you tune in to your body's signals, so you can identify when it's hungry, tired, stressed, or in need of movement. When you listen to your body, you can better understand its needs and respond in a way that supports your weight loss goals.

For example, sometimes we eat because we feel tired or bored, not because we're hungry. By being more aware of your body's needs through mindfulness, you'll be able to recognize these patterns and make healthier decisions. Over time, you'll develop a stronger ability to respond to your body's cues with compassion, leading to a more balanced, intuitive approach to eating and movement.

- Incorporating Movement with Intention

The mind-body connection also plays a key role in movement and exercise. When you view physical activity through the lens of **mindfulness and intention**, you begin to move in a way that honors your body rather than pushing it through a rigid routine. Whether it's through somatic exercises, yoga, or simply walking, when you move with awareness, you reduce the risk of injury, alleviate stress, and experience a sense of joy in your movement.

When your movements are aligned with your mind, you're more likely to stick with an exercise routine because it feels like a form of self-care rather than a chore. The more you connect with your body, the more empowered you will feel to engage in activities that promote weight loss in a healthy, sustainable way.

Practices to Strengthen the Mind-Body Connection

To help you strengthen the mind-body connection, here are a few practices that you can incorporate into your daily routine:

1. **Body Scan Meditation**: This simple practice involves slowly scanning your body from head to toe, paying attention to how each area feels. It helps bring awareness to any areas of tension or discomfort and allows you to release stress physically and mentally.

2. **Mindful Eating**: Take time to eat without distractions. Focus on the taste, texture, and smell of your food, and pause between bites. This helps you connect with your body's hunger and fullness cues and avoid overeating.

3. **Movement with Awareness**: Whether it's yoga, somatic exercises, or walking, practice moving with awareness. Pay attention to how your body feels as you move, and avoid pushing yourself too hard. This creates a sense of harmony between your body and mind, making exercise feel more enjoyable and less like a task.

4. **Journaling**: Writing down your thoughts and feelings can help you become more aware of any limiting beliefs or emotional patterns that may be affecting your weight loss journey. Journaling about your progress, setbacks, and achievements helps you shift your mindset toward a positive, growth-oriented perspective.

CHAPTER 4: SOMATIC EXERCISE FOR INCREASING PHYSICAL STRENGTH

How Somatic Movements Enhance Core Strength

You are not alone if you have been experiencing difficulty with physical strength, particularly in your core. Many of us rely on traditional methods to develop our core strength, such as sit-ups, crunches, and weight lifting. While these exercises can be beneficial, they do not always account for the deeper, more underlying strength your body requires. Somatic movements, on the other hand, are game changers. These mindful, body-centered techniques help you connect with your muscles and movement patterns in ways that standard workouts often do not.

Understanding how your body moves as a whole, how your breath affects movement, and how your muscles work throughout daily chores are all important aspects of core strength. It's not just about how many crunches you can perform. In addition to addressing all of these issues, somatic exercises are highly successful in developing a solid, strong core that promotes physical vitality and weight loss.

The Core: More Than Just Abs

Let's clarify what we mean by "core" before getting into the mechanics of somatic motions. Many people assume that the core consists solely of the abdominal muscles, which are the part of the body that everyone wishes to tone. Although it includes the abs, your core is far more expansive. It consists of the muscles in your back, hips, and pelvis, which cooperate to give your body strength and stability. Almost every movement you do, whether you're dancing, moving groceries, or even just sitting at your desk, starts with your core. When your core is weak or disconnected, you may experience poor posture, discomfort, or even pain. By strengthening your core with somatic movements, you're building functional strength that supports everything you do, from everyday activities to more intense workouts.

What Are Somatic Movements?

Somatic movements focus on body awareness, mindfulness, and controlled, purposeful motion. They are designed to bring attention to the sensations in the body and how it moves through space. Unlike traditional exercises that often focus on repetition and intensity, somatic exercises encourage you to slow down and tune into your body, allowing you to move in ways that feel natural and effective.

For example, somatic exercises might involve slow, fluid movements that engage the whole body, such as pelvic tilts, spinal articulation, or gentle rotations. These exercises help you reconnect with your body's natural alignment and movement patterns, especially in the core area.

Proper posture, pelvic support, and spine stability are all made possible by the deep muscles of the core, which are activated by somatic movements. Because they mainly target the superficial abdominal muscles, typical exercises like crunches frequently overlook these muscles. A more comprehensive and long-lasting method of developing core strength is offered by somatic exercises, which focus on these deeper layers.

How Somatic Movements Enhance Core Strength

- Awareness of Alignment: One of the first steps in strengthening your core through somatic movement is developing awareness of your body's alignment. Many of us go through life without noticing how our posture affects our core stability. We might sit slumped at a desk or stand with our weight shifted to one side. Somatic practices help you become aware of these imbalances so you can correct them. By simply noticing your posture and how your body feels during movements, you start to engage the muscles of your core in a more efficient way.
- Breath-Body Connection: Breath is deeply tied to core strength. When we breathe deeply, especially into the diaphragm, it naturally engages the deep core muscles. Somatic movements often integrate breathwork to help you connect to your body and activate these muscles. For

instance, when you perform a gentle movement like a spinal roll or a pelvic tilt, focusing on your breath can help you activate your core muscles. Breathing deeply as you move helps to strengthen the diaphragm, which plays a key role in stabilizing the core. This is something that traditional exercises often overlook but is crucial for building a stable, functional core.

- Slow, Controlled Movements: Somatic exercises emphasize the quality of movement over quantity. By performing movements slowly and with control, you force your muscles to engage more deeply and effectively. When you move slowly, you give yourself time to focus on the muscles you're working, allowing them to activate properly. This slow, deliberate approach is especially beneficial for strengthening the deeper muscles of the core. For example, a simple slow reach of the arm overhead while maintaining a stable pelvis forces the core muscles to engage in a supportive and stabilizing manner, helping to build strength and control.

- Muscle Integration: Unlike traditional core exercises that may isolate specific muscles, somatic movements focus on integrating multiple muscle groups. By moving the body as a whole, rather than just focusing on one muscle group, somatic practices help your muscles work in harmony, which is essential for developing balanced strength. For instance, movements like hip circles or side stretches engage the core muscles, back, and legs simultaneously. This holistic approach not only strengthens the core but also improves the flexibility and mobility of the surrounding muscles, which support the core in its various functions.

- Releasing Tension and Tightness: Chronic tension and tightness in the body can limit your ability to engage the core effectively. Somatic exercises help to release this built-up tension, particularly in areas like the lower back and pelvis, which are key parts of the core. For example, gentle stretching and twisting movements can help to release tightness and improve the flexibility of the muscles surrounding your core. As you release this tension, you create more space for your core muscles to engage and strengthen, improving both mobility and stability.
- Functional Strength: Core strength isn't just about looking good or holding a plank for an extended period, it's about how your body functions in real-life situations. Somatic exercises focus on building functional strength that will serve you in daily activities. When your core is strong and stable, you're better able to lift objects safely, maintain good posture, and move with fluidity and grace. Through mindful somatic movements, you're training your body to be both strong and adaptable, which is essential for overall physical health and mobility.

How to Start Enhancing Core Strength with Somatic Movements

You don't need to do hours of intense exercise to strengthen your core, somatic movements are designed to be gentle, accessible, and effective. Here are a few exercises to get you started:

- Pelvic Tilts: Lying on your back with your knees bent, gently tilt your pelvis forward and backward, engaging your lower abdominal muscles. This helps to activate the deep core muscles and improve mobility in the pelvis.

- Spinal Rolls: While sitting or standing, slowly roll your spine down one vertebra at a time, then roll it back up, one vertebra at a time. This movement helps improve spinal alignment, mobility, and strengthens the muscles along your back and abdomen.

- Side Stretches: Stand tall and reach one arm overhead, leaning gently to the side to stretch through the torso. This opens up the muscles along your sides and helps engage the obliques, which are key components of the core.

- Breathwork: Lie on your back with one hand on your chest and one on your abdomen. As you breathe in, allow your abdomen to rise, engaging your diaphragm and deep core muscles. Exhale slowly, drawing your navel in toward your spine. Repeat this for several minutes to activate your deep core muscles and connect your breath to movement.

The Long-Term Benefits of a Strong Core

Somatic exercises that strengthen the core are beneficial for longevity, health, and function in addition to appearance. Your entire body is supported by a strong core, which facilitates daily tasks, enhances posture, and guards against injury. You'll have more physical freedom and energy as well as more body confidence as you develop internal strength. Somatic exercises improve your general well-being by enabling you to navigate life with elegance and strength.

Adding somatic exercises to your practice can help you develop a strong, robust core that will assist you in all facets of your life, not simply get a six-pack.

How Somatic Exercises Increase Functional Strength

What is Functional Strength?

Functional strength is about how your body moves in real-world situations. It's different from the kind of strength you might develop in the gym where exercises are often isolated to one muscle group at a time. In real life, your body needs to move holistically. Every time you squat to pick something up, reach for an item on a shelf, or twist to get into your car, you're using multiple muscle groups working together in coordinated motion. Functional strength trains your body to move efficiently, without unnecessary strain.

Consider raising a large, hefty object off the ground, for instance. Your legs, core, back, and even your balance and coordination all play a part in the task, not just your arms. By enabling you to use certain muscle groups efficiently, functional strength makes jobs like this simpler, safer, and more effective. It's the difference between laboriously carrying a heavy object and effortlessly doing so without giving it any thought.

How Somatic Exercises Increase Functional Strength

Somatic exercises are incredibly effective at increasing functional strength because they focus on body awareness, coordination, and full-body engagement. These exercises help you move in ways that reflect how your body naturally moves in everyday life, which is why they are so valuable. Rather than isolating muscles, somatic exercises strengthen the entire kinetic chain, from your feet all the way up to your shoulders. Here's how somatic exercises contribute to functional strength:

- **Improving Mobility and Flexibility:**

Functional strength isn't just about how strong you are; it's also about how well your muscles and joints move. Somatic exercises improve mobility and flexibility, allowing you to move more freely and with less discomfort. For example, exercises like hip circles or spinal articulation help release stiffness and increase the range of motion in your joints. This enhanced mobility makes everyday tasks like bending down or reaching up less taxing on your body.

The more mobile and flexible you are, the easier it becomes to move without resistance, reducing the risk of injury.

- **Engaging the Deep Core Muscles:**

Your core is essential for functional strength. Without a strong, stable core, it's difficult to perform most physical activities, whether it's carrying groceries or playing with your kids. Somatic exercises focus on activating your deep core muscles, including the muscles that stabilize your spine and pelvis. By engaging these muscles with mindful movement, you build a foundation of strength that supports your entire body. Whether it's performing a gentle pelvic tilt or a controlled spinal roll, these movements work to strengthen the core in a way that translates directly into real-life activities.

- **Enhancing Coordination and Balance:**

Functional strength isn't just about brute force; it's also about being able to coordinate your movements and maintain balance. Somatic exercises often include movements that challenge your balance, such as shifting weight from one leg to another or standing on one leg while performing a slow movement. These exercises help train your body to stay balanced and stable in various positions, improving your ability to walk, climb stairs, or even navigate through uneven terrain. Stronger balance and coordination make everyday tasks much easier, while also reducing the risk of falls and injury.

- **Building Mindful Movement Patterns:**

Somatic exercises teach you to move mindfully. When you focus on how your body feels in each movement, you develop a better understanding of how to move efficiently and without strain. This can be a game-changer when it comes to functional strength, because it helps you avoid unnecessary tension or awkward movements that could lead to injury. By practicing mindful movements, you create more fluid and natural motion, making everything from carrying a load to reaching for something easier and more effective.

- **Strengthening the Entire Body:**

One of the key principles of somatic exercises is the idea of whole-body engagement. Instead of isolating specific muscles, somatic movements involve your entire body, working together to create functional strength. For example, lunges or squats might incorporate the use of your legs, core, and upper body all at once, training your body to coordinate multiple muscle groups. This full-body engagement improves not just your strength but also your endurance and stability, which are essential for functional movement.

- **Reducing Tension and Improving Posture:**

Somatic exercises help release built-up tension in your body, especially in areas like your neck, shoulders, and lower back, which are prone to tightness. This release of tension improves your posture, allowing you to stand, sit, and move more comfortably. A strong, aligned posture is key to functional strength because it ensures that your muscles and joints are working optimally. Poor posture can lead to muscle imbalances, which in turn can cause pain or hinder your ability to perform everyday tasks. Through somatic practices, you can correct these imbalances and create a more efficient, strong posture.

- **Improving Breathing and Energy Flow:**

Breathing is an essential part of functional strength. The way you breathe during movement can either support or hinder your efforts. Somatic exercises often incorporate breathwork to ensure that your body is properly oxygenated, helping your muscles to perform at their best. When you breathe deeply and mindfully, you activate your diaphragm and core muscles, allowing for more effective movement and better energy flow throughout the body. This increased oxygenation enhances your overall stamina and strength, making physical activities less exhausting.

Why Somatic Exercises Are Ideal for Functional Strength

Because somatic workouts replicate real-life movement patterns, they are extremely effective at enhancing functional strength. They teach your body to move more effectively and mindfully rather than isolating particular muscle groups like traditional strength training routines do. Somatic exercises develop strength that is both useful and long-lasting by fortifying the entire kinetic chain. Not only are you becoming stronger, but you're also learning how to move confidently, fluidly, and easily in daily situations.

Functional strength is about feeling empowered in your own body, not just in the gym, but in every task you take in. Whether it's lifting a child, moving furniture, or simply getting out of bed without pain, somatic exercises help you to build the kind of strength that enhances your quality of life.

Starting Your Journey to Functional Strength

If you're new to somatic exercises, start with slow, mindful movements that help you tune in to your body. Begin with simple practices like gentle stretches, pelvic tilts, or spinal rolls. Focus on how your body feels as you move and gradually increase the range of motion as you build strength and mobility. Over time, you'll notice how your body becomes more stable, resilient, and capable in everyday situations.

CHAPTER 5: 28 DAYS NUTRITIONAL PLAN

This 28-day meals plan is intended to supplement the advantages of somatic workouts while giving the body the nutrients it needs for energy, weight loss, muscle regeneration, and general health. It is composed of full, nutrient-dense foods that will support your body's ability to heal, maintain energy, and burn fat more efficiently.

Guidelines for the Nutritional Plan:

- Stay Hydrated: Drink plenty of water throughout the day, especially before and after your somatic exercises. Hydration is key for muscle recovery and keeping your body energized.
- Prioritize Protein: Include high-quality proteins in your meals to support muscle repair and reduce hunger cravings.
- Healthy Fats: Healthy fats from sources like avocado, nuts, and olive oil will support energy levels and brain function.
- Complex Carbs: Choose whole grains like quinoa, oats, and brown rice to fuel your exercise routine and provide steady energy throughout the day.
- Incorporate Vegetables: Aim to fill half your plate with vegetables at every meal for maximum nutrients and fiber.

- Limit Processed Foods and Sugars: Avoid processed foods, sugary snacks, and refined carbs. Stick to whole, unprocessed foods as much as possible.

Weekly Overview:

Each week will have a distinct theme, with an emphasis on important nutrients for weight loss and somatic exercise recovery.

Week 1: Detox and Energize

The first week focuses on **cleaning up the diet**, reducing inflammation, and boosting energy. Fresh vegetables, lean proteins, and healthy fats are key.

- **Breakfast:**
  - Green Smoothie (spinach, kale, almond milk, chia seeds, banana, and protein powder)
  - Oatmeal with almonds, berries, and a teaspoon of chia seeds
- **Lunch:**
  - Grilled chicken salad with avocado, spinach, cucumber, and a lemon-olive oil dressing
  - Lentil soup with a side of mixed greens
- **Dinner:**

- o Baked salmon with roasted Brussels sprouts and sweet potato

  - o Stir-fried tofu with broccoli, bell peppers, and brown rice

- **Snack Ideas:**

  - o Apple with a handful of almonds

  - o Carrot sticks and hummus

Week 2: Strength and Recovery

During this week, we'll emphasize **protein-rich foods** to support muscle repair and recovery from the somatic exercises. Foods rich in omega-3s will also reduce inflammation.

- **Breakfast:**

  - o Scrambled eggs with spinach and mushrooms

  - o Greek yogurt with chia seeds, walnuts, and mixed berries

- **Lunch:**

  - o Grilled turkey or chicken breast with quinoa and a mixed vegetable salad

  - o Veggie-packed chili with kidney beans, bell peppers, and zucchini

- **Dinner:**

  - o Grilled shrimp with cauliflower rice and steamed asparagus o Baked chicken thighs with roasted carrots and quinoa

- **Snack Ideas:**

    o Handful of mixed nuts (almonds, walnuts, cashews)

    o Hard-boiled egg with a sprinkle of sea salt

Week 3: Fat Burning and Metabolism Boost

The third week focuses on boosting **fat-burning** metabolism with high-fiber foods, healthy fats, and green vegetables. The goal is to continue the momentum of weight loss while maintaining energy for somatic exercise.

- **Breakfast:**

    o Chia pudding made with coconut milk, topped with berries

    o Scrambled eggs with avocado and a side of tomatoes

- **Lunch:**

    o Grilled salmon with roasted Brussels sprouts and avocado

    o Sweet potato and black bean salad with a cilantro-lime dressing

- **Dinner:**

    o Zucchini noodles with grilled chicken and a tomato-based sauce

    o Roasted turkey with sautéed spinach and steamed broccoli

- **Snack Ideas:**

- Cucumber and carrot sticks with guacamole

- Greek yogurt with flaxseeds

Week 4: Maintenance and Nourishment

In the final week, the meal plan will help **balance your nutrition**, making sure you're fueling your body with the right foods to sustain energy, support muscle recovery, and continue your weight loss journey.

- **Breakfast:**

    - Smoothie with almond milk, protein powder, spinach, frozen berries, and peanut butter

    - Scrambled tofu with sautéed kale and avocado

- **Lunch:**

    - Grilled chicken breast with quinoa, avocado, and a side of roasted sweet potatoes

    - Vegan Buddha bowl with chickpeas, roasted veggies, and tahini dressing

- **Dinner:**

    - Grilled shrimp with a kale and quinoa salad, topped with olive oil and lemon dressing

- Baked cod with roasted cauliflower and a side of sautéed mushrooms

- **Snack Ideas:**

  - Celery with almond butter

  - A small handful of walnuts or mixed nuts

Additional Nutritional Tips to Support Somatic Exercise:

Pre-Exercise Fuel:

- A small snack with healthy carbohydrates and protein 30 minutes before exercise can help boost energy levels. For example, a banana with a tablespoon of peanut butter or a slice of whole-grain toast with avocado.

Post-Exercise Recovery:

- After your somatic session, aim to eat a meal that includes **protein and carbohydrates** to aid in muscle recovery. A post-workout meal might include a small serving of **chicken with brown rice** or **Greek yogurt with some berries** to help replenish glycogen stores and repair muscles.

Hydration:

- Always hydrate before, during, and after exercise. You might also add **electrolytes** into your water (especially if you've had a particularly intense somatic session) to replenish lost minerals and prevent dehydration.

A demonstration day for weight loss and somatic exercise support:

Breakfast:

- Scrambled eggs with spinach and avocado

- Green tea

Lunch:

- Grilled chicken salad with mixed greens, avocado, cucumber, and a vinaigrette dressing

Snack:

- A handful of mixed nuts and a cup of herbal tea

Dinner:

- Baked salmon with roasted Brussels sprouts, quinoa, and a side of steamed kale

Snack (if needed):

- Apple with almond butter or a small piece of dark chocolate (70% or higher)

CONCLUSION

Starting on a path to greater health and weight loss does not have to be intimidating or difficult. You've learned how to connect with your body in a more attentive, purposeful way by practicing somatic exercises, which strengthen it, reduce stress, and improve mobility.

When combined with a balanced, healthy 28-day food plan, you now have the skills to fuel your body, improve recovery, and support your weight loss objectives. Keep in mind that this journey is about more than simply physical change; it's also about learning more about who you are and what your body requires. Somatic techniques respect your body's natural rhythms while enabling you to move more easily, experience less pain, and develop functional strength. In addition to losing weight, a nutrient-dense diet can help you feel more in tune with your body and more energized and refreshed.

The path ahead requires self-love, perseverance, and patience. Have faith that long-lasting change is occurring from the inside out as you continue to integrate somatic workouts and a nutritious diet into your daily routine. By completing these actions, you are creating a stronger, healthier, and more connected version of yourself. You can achieve your transformation if you persevere.